Table of Contents:

Chapter 7: From One to Unlimited

Helping Your Lover Find Your G-Spot
Gentle Anal Activity
Moving on to Conventional Intercourse

Chapter 8: Additional Advice
Variety Spices Things Up
Communication is Crucial
Keep Expectations Reasonable

Conclusion

Introduction

Intimate desires are among the oldest and most natural ingrained features humans possess. They're right up there with hunger, thirst and exhaustion. We are driven to satisfy these urges just as we are to eat, drink, sleep and protect our loved ones.

Unfortunately, the majority of women express frustration with the intimate portion of their lives. This often stems from a lack of variety. That one depriving factor can be driven by fear of experiencing uncharted territory or a simple lack of knowledge of the potential within their own bodies.

Most women are capable of achieving orgasm; furthermore, virtually all those who can reach one are able to take this a few steps further. This leads to having several during a single intimate session. It may take a little practice at first, but it's well within your reach.

Men and women alike suffer from a widespread misconception that having an orgasm during the actual act of intercourse is the norm. It's not; in fact, only about a fourth of women actually reach this point during conventional intercourse. If you're one of those, you are far from alone.

There's nothing wrong with you or your individual anatomy. All you need is a little push in the right direction to begin experiencing a much more exciting and satisfying sex life. With the right education, advice and encouragement, you can become one of the few who enjoys consistently explosive encounters whether alone or with a companion.

Chapter 1: The Secret Within

While the full reason women are able to have multiple orgasms remains somewhat of a mystery, experts agree the lion's share of the secret simply lies in the female anatomy. Though men tend to become aroused and reach their climax quickly, their sole center of attraction is the penis. Once a man arrives at the point of orgasm, his experience is typically over, and he needs anywhere from a couple of hours to a few days to build back up to another state of readiness.

Women, on the other hand, have a few advantages in this respect. The female body holds more than one key area allowing for full arousal. At the same time, those regions contain thousands more nerves than the tip of the penis. These two aspects mean women are able to experience continuous arousal and have the potential for far more climaxes without any interruption between them. That is, of course, if the right techniques are used.

Chapter 2: An Anatomy Lesson

You're probably aware of the existence of various erogenous zones, and these are crucial to sexual enjoyment. Three different types of these areas have been discovered, and each plays its own role in reaching your climax. Knowing those zones can be a big help in getting the most of out of your intimate encounters.

Tertiary Erogenous Zones:

These are the least sensitive of the relevant areas, but they're still important. These are the areas you or your partner should consider focusing on in the early stages of your encounter because they basically help build suspense. The tertiary areas include:

- Arms
- Legs
- Chest

Secondary Erogenous Zones:

Once the tertiary zones have received some attention, it's time to move on to the secondary zones. These aren't the true hot spots, but they are more sensitive than their previous counterparts. Again, they help heighten the positive type of tension ultimately leading to the climax. The secondary zones are:

- Hands
- Feet
- Neck
- Ears
- Breasts

Primary Erogenous Zones:

Those previous zones are simply segues to reaching the primary areas of the female body. The primary erogenous zones are vital to achieving an orgasm in the first place. They are far more sensitive than other areas of the body. These involve:

- Lips
- Nipples
- Genitals
- Anus

Beginning with the tertiary erogenous zones and working your way up to the primary ones, you can expand greatly upon your excitement by slowly inciting arousal. Think of it like reading a book. You could certainly pick up a novel and flip straight to the ending. You'd know how the story comes to a close, but you wouldn't have any context surrounding that point. You might gain a little satisfaction that way, but it couldn't come close to the complete fulfillment of taking your time and working your way up to the final point.

Chapter 3: The Art of Discovery

The previously mentioned erogenous zones are just the most common ones. Everyone is different. For you, it could be your partner kissing the bends of your legs, caressing your lower abdomen or sliding a hand down your rib cage or along your inner thighs that sends shivers through your body.

There's nothing wrong with being an individual, so the key is experimentation. In fact, many couples stumble upon their own unique hot spots completely by accident. Be sure to pay attention during your encounters to uncover what works best for you.

Chapter 4: Delving Deeper into the Experience

Now that you know the basics of the feminine anatomy, you can explore things a bit further. Amidst the primary erogenous zones are a few key areas to discover. The genitals alone hold their own hidden potential. Developing awareness of these aspects can help you expand from an occasional single orgasm to regular multiple climaxes.

The Clitoris:

This is likely to be the most sensitive area of your entire body; in fact, far more women are able to achieve orgasm via clitoral stimulation than through conventional intercourse. If you fall into this category, you're definitely not alone. In case you have yet to understand exactly where your clitoris lies, here's how to locate it:

- Find your vaginal opening.
- Move upward a bit to your labia.
- Separate the folds of your inner labia.

The small bud of tender skin at the top of those folds where they meet will be your clitoris. This spot alone holds almost twice the number of nerve endings as the tip of the male penis and tends to make it the best area to focus on to achieve an initial orgasm. Of course, the experience doesn't end there.

The G-Spot:

Many have heard of this seemingly magical area, but not many understand what it is. It's actually located inside the vagina and can also be used to reach your climax. These are the steps to finding your G-spot:

- Insert your finger in your vagina.
- Curl your finger slightly toward the front of your body.
- Slide your finger along the forward wall of the vagina, usually about 1 to 3 inches from its opening.

You should find a pronounced lump of soft tissue, and that would be your G-spot. This, too, has a number of sensitive nerve endings, making it equally important in the multi-orgasmic venture.

The Anterior Fornix Erotic Zone:

This isn't as commonly heard of as the G-spot, and it can be a little more difficult to find, but it's also quite receptive to touch. You may actually need some help unearthing this particular spot though this is how it's done:

- Find your G-spot.
- Slide your finger, or have your partner do this, deeper along the front side of the vagina.
- The AFE should be located near your cervix.

Since it's much further inside the vagina than your G-spot, the AFE is sometimes elusive. Penile penetration or a curved vibrator may be needed in this case; however, you'll typically know when you've found it.

The Anus:

The skin surrounding your anus and running from your vaginal opening back additionally has plenty of nerve endings. Massaging this area can often induce climax, but in some instances, a little more effort may be required.

Penetration of the anus is sometimes enough to send a pleasurable shock through your body, yet this can also be an outside portal for G-spot stimulation.

Putting it All Together:

Those are the intricacies of the primary female erogenous zones. A little time and attention given to either of these will generally bring on a climax. Moving methodically from one to another tends to elicit those serial orgasms you may be interested in experiencing.

Chapter 5: Finding Your Own Way

Though few scenarios can compare to sharing sexual experiences with a partner, learning exactly what gets you most aroused is often best accomplished alone. While you can't exactly kiss your own neck or try out other techniques your partner could help with, you can test a number of strategies by yourself in the privacy of your own home. When you find what is most effective for you, you can then pass this interesting information along to a playmate.

Set the Scene:

As is the case with just about any task, you're not going to get much accomplished if distractions abound. You'll need to save your lone wolf endeavors until a time when you can truly be alone. This may be after a roommate has gone out for the evening or when the kids are sound asleep. There's no shame in calling in sick, so you can take a day off work if necessary.

Lock the bedroom door, turn off the lights and your phone, and completely clear your mind. If you'd like, you could light some candles for ambience and turn on some soft music. This is completely up to you; do what makes you feel comfortable.

Few people will tell you this, but when you're planning to do this type of exploration, be sure not to eat a large meal beforehand. You don't want to be so hungry you can't concentrate, but you also don't want to stuff yourself. If you do, you're bound to feel bloated and uncomfortable from the beginning. Then, you'll be more likely to take a nap than to enjoy finding out what gets you going.

Once you're ready to begin, lie down and get comfortable. Don't worry about how you look at the moment; remember, you're alone. If warm fuzzy socks and a worn out t-shirt make you feel cozy and secure, go for it.

Ease into the Experience:

When you're with a partner, it's important to work your way up to the main event. The same is true when you're flying solo. You may want to start off by getting your mind in the mood. Let your fantasies run amok, imagining an experience you've had in the past or one you'd like to have in the future. Daydream like this for a while until you're ready to take it a step further.

From there, you could consider rubbing your breasts and nipples or caressing your hips and inner thighs to further build the anticipation. Your fingers can be your most useful tools in self exploration, so once you've gotten yourself a little more excited, you can move on to your genital area. Try lightly penetrating your vagina or anus and massaging the surrounding skin. This would be a great time to experiment with your G-spot as well. Put various amounts of pressure and diverse angles to the test to figure out what feels best.

When the right time comes, you can focus on your most sensitive area: the clitoris. Gently rubbing along

14

its sides or across the area immediately above your clitoris can provide intense stimulation, but adding greater speed or more pressure may be needed. If you want or need it, direct clitoral attention can also be helpful. This may be less comfortable and pleasurable if the skin is dry, so use lubricants or saliva to make the experience go more smoothly.

Taking it up a Notch:

If you feel you've mastered conventional self exploration, or you've grown bored with such techniques, you haven't reached the end of the road. Consider introducing yourself to certain toys. Vibrators are available in an array of sizes, shapes, materials and speed options. These are common vessels for those who are ready to ramp up their efforts.

External and internal stimulation can be achieved using these devices. They tend to be very accommodating when it comes to finding your G-spot and anterior fornix erotic zone. Since a number of women find reaching and stimulating these areas on their own, such a tool may be vital to learning as much as possible through self exploration.

Similar to the initial stages of discovering what turns you on, trying out these tools on different areas of

15

your body using varying techniques can go a long way toward discovering your innermost desires. Keep in mind, the world of intimate toys is vast, so consider all the options out there.

Since the anal area is among the key pleasure zones, you might be interested in devices geared toward this region. Though starting off this type of exploration with your pinky factor might be your best course of action, anal beads also come in a range of sizes. Start off small, and work your way up if you enjoy it.

Anal plugs can also be used, and they, too, are offered in varying diameters. When it comes to anal exploration, be sure to use ample amounts of lubricant. Not doing so is a very common mistake and one of the primary reasons women see this as such a painful experience.

Chapter 6: Sharing the Journey

The best way to find just what arouses you most may be to explore your options alone, but getting your playmate involved has a tendency to bring much more to the table. For starters, your partner can work on your tertiary and secondary erogenous zones much more easily than you can. Secondly, oral interaction is only possible with another individual.

Last, but not least, your partner can add the element of surprise. You know where your hands and toys are going, but partners have minds of their own. You never know what might happen next. Though you may have discovered much of what turns you on at this point, you could also learn a lot from that little hint of the unexpected.

Keep All the Vital Areas in Mind:

As mentioned previously, don't jump right to your primary erogenous zones; have your lover proceed slowly and gently at first. Your partner should start out by caressing or kissing your arms, legs and chest, perhaps between or along the outer edges of your breasts. This helps get your mind and body focused on the entire experience.

After both of you become more immersed in the encounter, it's time to move along to the secondary zones. A brief foot massage may be in order at this point, followed by caressing your palms. Holding hands with fingers interlocked while your partner uses lips and tongue to target your neck, ears and breasts then serves to intensify your desire. Once this has been accomplished, it's time to concentrate on other concerns.

Zeroing in on the Primary Zones:

Following the initial, less immediate stages of foreplay, the primary erogenous zones can enter the picture. Targeting the nipples with the lips, tongue and hands will more than likely heighten your awareness as a prelude to fixating on your genital area. Your clitoris is your pleasure center, but in line with the entire experience, it's important to build suspense.

Clitoral stimulation is typically the easiest path to your climax, yet a number of strategies can be used to reach that point. Many find oral encounters to be most satisfying if their partner carries this out appropriately. No specifically right or wrong tactics exist here; it all depends on what you find most gratifying.

A Few Helpful Oral Techniques:

Numerous women find absolutely no satisfaction through oral sex; in fact, some even come to dread this experience because their partners carry out the process too vigorously. It's important to start out slowly and gently. Commonly known as teasing, this is often the secret to ensuring a woman gets the most out of her partner's oral efforts. The following tips can be helpful in easing into an encounter of this sort.

- Slide the tongue lightly along the outer and inner labia in long, slow motions.

- Place the tongue flat against the skin between the anus and the vagina, licking up toward the clitoris.
- Move along to vaginal penetration using the tongue.
- Gently suck on the clitoris; alternately, lick this area with the tip of the tongue.

After beginning slowly, you can gradually work your way up to increased speed and pressure. Some find this is all they need to reach their initial orgasm. Others simply can't achieve a climax from such techniques. If not, the hands and fingers will become essential.

Proceeding From Oral to Manual:

When it comes to switching over to manual provocation, your accomplice can use the techniques you uncovered during self exploration. Another useful move is to have your partner place a hand against your genitals and press the palm against your vulva. Applying different finger motions, both externally and internally, adds variation to this portion of your encounter.

All this clitoral stimulation is bound to lead to an orgasm, but this can be an intense experience. It's also going to leave your clitoris and its surroundings extremely sensitive. To continue focusing on this region could lead to more pain than pleasure. This is where your alternative erogenous areas come into play and is also your gateway to a string of serial orgasms.

Chapter 7: From One to Unlimited

Once you reach that initial climax, your entire genital area is going to be far more sensitive. This means you've set your mind and body up to be more receptive to further orgasmic opportunities. As the second most sensitive component of your body, as well as one the easier aspects to locate and reach, you may want to have your partner focus on your G-spot next while giving your clitoris a bit of a break.

Helping Your Lover Find Your G-Spot:

This can't typically be reached easily with the tongue. If your partner happens to be able to make contact with your G-spot orally, they may not be able to place enough pressure on it to have much of an impact. The fingers have been found most effective here. One or two fingers can be inserted into your vagina to feel for this area. Your guidance and direction may be needed if your partner is unfamiliar with your particular G-spot or the concept in general.

If you're concerned that you've never had an orgasm through this type of action before, don't be. Bear in mind, the previous stimulation and resulting climax will render other areas more vulnerable to attention. A few moments of slightly persuasive stroking or pressing force on your G-spot could easily lead into the second event in a series of pinnacles.

Gentle Anal Activity:

Your anal area can be incorporated though you may want to proceed carefully. This is an especially tender region and should be treated as such. If you choose to allow anal penetration, have your partner start off with a pinky finger and ease it inside very slowly. Also be sure to implement plenty of lubricant. If your body produces excess amounts naturally during your previous climaxes, this can assist your playmate; otherwise, synthetic options will work well.

Many women find achieving orgasm during anal activity to be difficult, but since you're already more stimulated and receptive, a positive outcome could be reached. Anal penetration could also be another pathway to G-spot stimulation. Either way, yet another climax could come from this area.

Moving on to Conventional Intercourse:

Less than 25 percent of women actually experience climax during intercourse, leaving millions leading less than fulfilling sex lives. With those thousands of nerves centralized in the female genital region already on edge from pre-intercourse orgasms, this could change as well. Begin with achieving at least one orgasm during foreplay.

This could lead to unprecedented satisfaction while you're involved in the actual act of intercourse. If it doesn't happen for you, don't be discouraged. You could always have your partner return concentration to other areas afterward.

Chapter 8: Additional Advice

First of all, don't be afraid to experiment both alone and with someone else. Find those areas that provide you with the most stimulation and then share them with your playmate. Discovering new strategies together can be just as enticing. Just be sure your cohort is comfortable with any suggestions you offer; if not, neither of you will get as much enjoyment out of the experience.

Variety Spices Things Up:

Try different routines and positions. Though finding the combination of techniques that bring about your first few experiences with serial orgasms can be exciting, holding yourself and your partner to this exact series of activities can become stale just like anything else in your life. You could also introduce various toys into your shared love life if your partner is open to such an idea. Variety is the spice of life, and it can certainly enhance your intimate encounters.

Communication is Crucial:

Your companion may have learned some of the things you like and dislike over time, but no one can read your mind. If something a partner is doing feels good but could be better, convey this to them. Likewise, gently let it be known if something hurts you or just isn't having any positive effect. Don't be hateful or derogatory; just offer a little helpful direction.

You could do this verbally, by guiding your playmate's hand or by using your own hands to point them in the right direction. Not only will it help make the experience more fulfilling for you, it'll also assist in boosting confidence and reducing inhibition for your partner.

Keep Expectations Reasonable:

If you go into a rendezvous doubting you'll find fulfillment, that's probably going to be the end result.

At the same time, if you engage in contact anticipating ten climaxes and only experience one or two, you're bound to be disappointed. Enter your encounters with positivity, but don't let your expectations get out of hand. Enjoy every moment of the jaunt leading up to your first orgasm, and the rest is just icing on the cake.

Conclusion

Studies reveal 75 percent of women are dissatisfied with their sex lives; in contrast, experts insist an estimated 98 percent of women are capable of achieving an orgasm. These same experts state any woman who is able to have one is also capable of reaching multiple climaxes over the course of a single encounter.

The key lies not in individual physiology, but in your level of understanding of how your mind and body work. A little knowledge of the many techniques you could use to help you along the way doesn't hurt either.

As a final reminder, here are some of the important things to remember leading up to and during your intimate scenarios.

Do:

- Keep your erogenous zones in mind.

- Ease into encounters by starting out with your tertiary erogenous zones and working your way up to the primary ones.
- Concentrate on all your possible hot spots rather than only one.
- Try self exploration before you share intimate contact with someone else.
- Relax and enjoy the experience for what it is regardless of the number of orgasms you have.
- Calmly and understandingly communicate your likes and dislikes to your partner.
- Make variation a priority.
- Be open to trying new positions and techniques.

Don't:

- Let distractions detract from an experience.
- Get stuck in a sexual rut simply because you find a combination of strategies that works for you.
- Limit yourself by having unreasonable expectations from an encounter.
- Rush to get to the primary erogenous zones.
- Make each rendezvous a race to see how many climaxes you can achieve.

- Become discouraged if you don't succeed in achieving serial orgasms during your first few attempts.

Once you reach your first pinnacle during an encounter, your mind and body will be more susceptible to others that could follow. After you first find your ability to have numerous climaxes during a single escapade, this capacity grows stronger and comes more easily with each experience. The potential for serial orgasms hinges on continual but varied stimulation of your entire genital region.

Using the advice and techniques provided, you could progress from a single orgasm during an occasional intimate session to multiple explosions every time you're at bat. Join the few have unleashed their full climactic potential. Become the serial orgasmic woman you were destined to be!